Homemade Laundry Detergent

30 Recipes of Safe DIY Detergent

Table of Contents

Introduction

I would first like to thank and congratulate you on downloading *"Homemade Laundry Detergent."* You will be so glad that you decided to begin to use homemade laundry detergents for a variety of reasons. In this day and age we must try and come up with ways that we can make our budget stretch further, using homemade natural laundry detergents will help you to accomplish this.

Not only is store bought laundry detergents and soaps expensive but they are also filled with all kinds of harsh chemicals, which will not only damage items of clothing but also can cause skin irritations. We all need to use laundry detergents to clean our clothes, they are a must in daily life, but we do not have to use expensive store bought chemical filled types of detergent. Instead you can feel a lot better in knowing your homemade laundry detergent is a natural product that will be gentle on your clothing items and skin as well as your pocket book!

Chapter 1. Our Need for Laundry Detergent

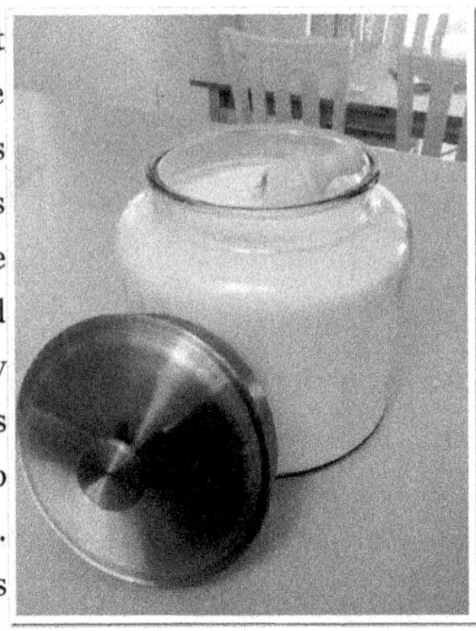

Laundry detergent is one of the items that most households contain. We need to wash our clothes so we need to have laundry detergents to do so. Clothing is the most important accessory of man, hence it is important that we clean our clothing. It can be challenging to keep clothes clean so having a good quality laundry detergent is important. Laundry detergent is one of the most important cleaning items included in most homes. Laundry detergent is used to wash articles of clothing made from various materials. Using laundry detergent helps us to clean our clothes more easily along with water.

Laundry detergents are a mixture of chemical compounds which are similar to soap in action but are less affected by hard water. Laundry detergents today contain alkylbenzenesulfonates that are highly effective in cleaning our laundry and are also more biodegradable.

There is often on average two loads of laundry to be washed per day for even a small family. The washing is never ending for most households, there is always something that needs to be washed such as bed sheets, baby clothes, towels, under garments, they will contain various types of stains, will have dead skin cells collecting on them etc. Helping to keep your clothes clean are the surfactants found in your laundry detergent. Many people today are starting to turn away from using commercial detergents which are loaded with various chemicals and instead are turning to using natural homemade laundry detergents.

Homemade Detergents

The best way for you to increase the life of your articles of clothing and to keep your skin from becoming irritated due to harsh chemicals in store bought laundry detergents is to start using homemade laundry detergent. You can buy all the ingredients you will need to make homemade laundry detergent in the stores, and they are not costly. You are going to be pleasantly surprised at the great quality and eco-friendly homemade laundry detergents you will be able to prepare for a very low cost. The three basic ingredients you will need is borax, washing soda, and naphtha soap or bar soap that you can easily prepare laundry detergents with. You can find these ingredients in the aisles where the laundry detergents are. You can even buy these products online. More and more people are turning towards using homemade laundry detergent for their clothing.

If you want your laundry detergent to have a nice scent then you can simply add some of your favorite essential oil to the detergent in order to enhance its fragrance. There are no chemicals in homemade laundry detergent such as chlorine, phosphates etc. There is no danger in using homemade detergents to the health of humans as well as the environment. Homemade detergents do not contain synthetic perfumes or dyes so they are also safe for people who have allergies to commercial detergents.

Homemade Detergent is Easy to Make

The great news is that it will only take you about 15-20 minutes to make your homemade laundry detergent that will be good for a month's use. You will find it easy to acquire the ingredients needed to begin to make your own laundry detergent. Most grocery stores will supply these products in their laundry supply section. You can also order them cheaply online as well from online suppliers of these items. You can feel good in knowing that the supplies you will need to make your own homemade laundry detergent will be easy to obtain.

You will find that you can quickly begin to make your own homemade laundry detergent in no time. Using homemade laundry detergents will make your clothing look fresh, clean and will be suds free after every wash, all this for a lot less money than you would spend on liquid detergent in the shops.

Homemade Laundry Detergents Advantages

- **They Are Safe**—By using natural and simple ingredients you can make your own homemade laundry detergents that will not irritate your skin. Making your own homemade detergents will assure you that there is no harmful chemicals being added to them.

- **Prevents Water Pollution**—Most of the detergents offered in the market are filled with phosphates which are causing algal blooms when it reaches the water body and it destroys the quality of the water in the bodies of water. Homemade laundry detergent does not contain phosphates or any other harsh chemicals and are non-polluting.

- **They Are Less Costly**—Homemade laundry detergents are much cheaper than branded detergents available on the market. You can save lots of money by using homemade laundry detergent. You can make quality liquid detergents, but their cost of production is very low compared to store bought detergents.

- **Earning Money**—You may even decide to earn some extra money by preparing homemade laundry detergents for friends and family members who also want to use environmentally friendly products.

- **Recycling Plastics**—When you are making the laundry detergents at your home, you will be avoiding the large plastic containers used for branded laundry detergents. You will begin to recycle your plastic containers by reusing them over and over to hold your homemade laundry detergent in.

- **They Work**—Even though homemade laundry detergents will not have the lather that commercial detergents do because of the absence of phosphates, they will still work just as effectively as the branded detergents when it comes to cleaning your clothing.

- **Storage**—You can store your homemade liquid detergent easily at home. It can easily be stored in plastic water bottles. Your homemade laundry detergent will last you a long time, you can even think of storing enough to do you for a year.

- **Create Scent Needed**—To add a nice scent to your laundry detergents you can add in some of your favorite essential oil.

- **Freezing The Liquid**—You can also decide to freeze your laundry detergent if you are making a large batch of it. You can then store it for a long time without the contents spoiling. You can store homemade laundry detergent using ice cube trays. When you want to use them all you need to do is to add a cube to your laundry load.

Chapter 2. Step by Step Procedure to Prepare Homemade Detergent

Making your own natural homemade laundry detergent is really not a difficult task, but one that is beneficial in numerous ways making it well worth the effort. When mixing the ingredients you want to make sure that you combine them properly so that you will have the best homemade laundry detergent that works well and is cost effective at the same time. People are becoming more and more fed 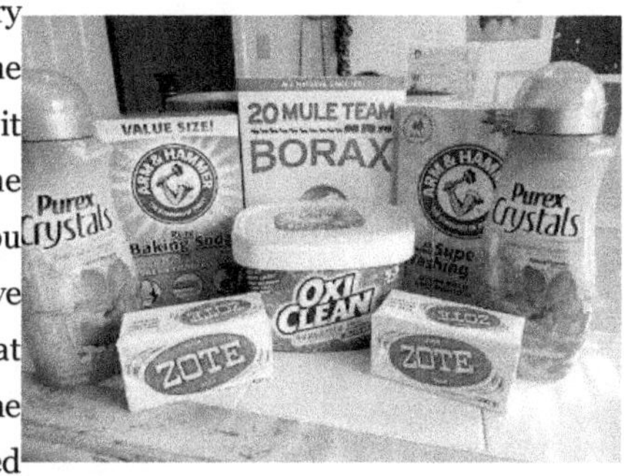 up with the high costs of so many items such as the high costs of commercial laundry detergents. This is a great driving factor for many to decide that they are going to start making their own homemade laundry detergent that will be low cost but effective in cleaning their clothing.

Many people are using the time tested and popular formulations to prepare homemade quality laundry detergent for literally pennies. Many believe that the time tested formula of homemade laundry detergent works far better at cleaning their clothes compared to the over-priced high quality commercial laundry detergents. The following is the simple and time tested formula used to make great quality homemade laundry detergent.

Ingredients You Will Need

Below are the important ingredients that you will need in order to make quality homemade laundry detergent.

- 1 cup of washing soda (make sure it is washing soda and not baking soda)

- 1 cup of any bar soap (choose one that is pure and natural for best results)

- 1/2 cup of borax

- 3 gallons of water

- Containers to store your laundry detergent (make sure that they come with lids)

- 1 pot for boiling your soapy water

- 1 large wooden spoon to stir

- 1 grater to grate the bar of soap

Step by Step Preparations

The following are the easy to follow step-by-step procedures that you will need to do to make your homemade laundry detergent. Follow these instructions and you will have your homemade laundry detergent in no time!

1. Place your grated pieces of soap into a bowl and then fill the bowl with water so that it completely submerges the soap.

2. Mix the soap in the water so that it develops into a soapy solution. You need to put this solution into a pot and boil it for a few minutes so that the soap gets completely melted so there is no bits of soap pieces floating about.

3. Another method you can use to prepare this soap solution is to first boil 4 cups of water in a pot on high. Once water is boiling, reduce the heat to a simmer. Add in the grated soap. Add soap into water in small quantities to make sure that the soap is all getting dissolved. Use wooden spoon to stir the soap while preparing. You need to make sure there are no soapy bits left but make sure it is all melted. The solution will look like an off white color.

4. Add into this solution a cup of washing soda and stir well using a wooden spoon. To avoid it from frothing too much gently stir it.

5. Next you will need to add in a cup of borax, mixing well with the wooden spoon to make sure it is well blended.

6. If you feel that using borax is too harsh then you can avoid it. Keep in mind that it does do a good cleaning job on clothes and also will leave clothing smelling fresh. I would suggest that you use at least half a cup of borax in your solution mixture.

7. It is important that you cook your mixture once again to make sure that it is melted completely. Do not bring it to a boil just warm it up and stir with wooden spoon. Cook it on simmer long enough so that all the ingredients are well blended. You should be left with a smooth creamy texture in your solution.

8. Now that it is a creamy solution it is now time for you to transfer it into your laundry soap containers. It would be a good idea to store it in gallon containers if you can.

9. Scoop the solution out of your pot using a measuring cup and fill up your containers. Do fill containers but just add in 3 to 4 cups of your creamy solution.

10. Now you need to add some hot water into the containers. Pour water in to container so that it is half full. Leave the top half of container empty. This will allow you to add more water if the solution becomes thicker or hardens.

11. Shake container with lid on so that the mix is well blended with added water.

12. Once the water is properly mixed with the solution allow the container to sit overnight.

13. The next morning you will find that the soap solution in your container has formed a big gooey substance. No worries this means that your homemade laundry detergent making process is on the right track.

14. Now, you have to break the gooey substance with a long wooden spoon. Once you break it you need to add some additional hot water just a bit from the top of the container.

15. Give container a good shake with lid on once again. It will turn into a rich creamy textured solution. This is how you make your own homemade laundry detergent for pennies.

16. There is no hard rules stating that your laundry detergent must have a certain amount of thickness. It does not matter if your homemade detergent is runny or thick it will work well for you as a natural homemade laundry detergent. As you get more experienced making your own laundry detergent you will figure out how much water to add to get the right thickness you desire in your detergent etc.

17. To add a bit of a fragrance to your laundry detergent you can also add a fragrance booster or essential oil of your choice to give your clothes a nice fresh clean smell.

18. Your detergent's thickness will depend on how much water you add to your solution as well as the type of soap you have used in the making of it. It could have a jell-o like consistency or it could be watery. All you have to do is to give it a stir and you are ready to use it.

19. Using a measuring cup measure out the amount of detergent that you want to use in your wash. It is ideal to use one cup of homemade laundry detergent per load.

20. You will soon find that your homemade laundry detergent is just as good if not better than any of the commercial quality laundry detergents on the market. What is really great is you can make your homemade detergent for pennies, making it very cheap to keep your clothes clean. Basically you will get nine scoops of homemade laundry detergent for the same cost as one scoop of quality commercial laundry detergents.

Chapter 3. Additional Homemade Laundry Detergent Recipes

1. *"Green" All Natural Laundry Detergent*
Ingredients:

- 1 bar of soap

- 1 cup of Oxi-Clean

- 2 cups of baking soda

- 1/2 cup of borax

- 1/2 box of washing soap

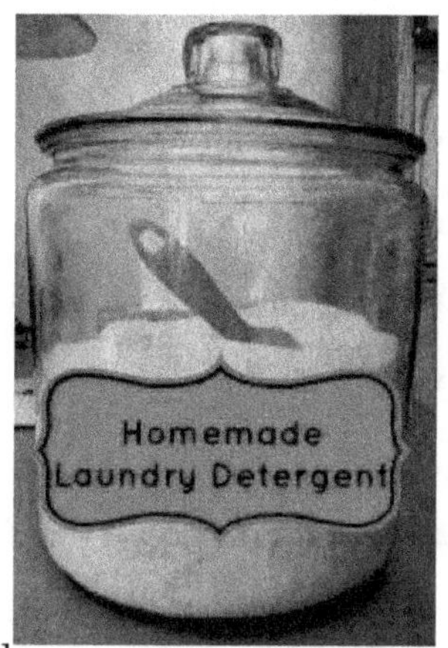

Directions:

Shred up the soap until it looks more like a powder. Add
and mix all of your ingredients and there you have some wonderful homemade "green"
laundry detergent.

2. *Vinegar-Based Laundry Powder*

Using this vinegar-based laundry powder will get your clothes clean without using any nasty chemicals. It will also help to neutralize unpleasant odors. If you are not fond of the aroma of vinegar do not worry it will evaporate quickly.

Ingredients:

- 1/2 cup of washing soda

- 1/2 cup of baking soda

- 1/8 cup of liquid Castile soap

- 1/2 cup of white vinegar

Directions:

In a large mixing bowl add in your Castile soap. Add in the washing soda and stir gently with wooden spoon. Stir until the mixture is well blended. Now, add in the baking soda and mix well. Slowly pour in the vinegar into the soap mix and continue to gently stir. It will develop a paste-like consistency before it gradually turns to a powder. Allow the mix to set for 30 minutes. Transfer it into a container with a tight sealing lid. Use 1 cup of vinegar-based laundry powder per load.

3. Homemade Laundry Soap Cubes

These are wonderful and simple to make laundry cubes—all you need to do is to toss two cubes into each load of your laundry. Any simple dry natural laundry detergent works well.

Ingredients:

- 3 to 4 cups of dry laundry detergent

- 1 spray bottle filled with white vinegar

Directions:

Add the dry laundry detergent into a mixing bowl and begin to spray it with white vinegar, stirring it constantly. Spray detergent until it is just moist enough to stick together when you squeeze small amount in your hand. Press this mixture firmly into ice cube tray, use one tablespoon per cube. Allow the cubes to air dry overnight, then remove them from ice cube tray. Store them in a plastic container.

4. *Simple Dry Laundry Detergent*

It only takes minutes to prepare this laundry detergent, with very little cleanup involved. Use your choice of natural soap, such as the popular Castile, or Ivory or your own homemade natural soap.

Ingredients:

- 1 cup of washing soda
- 1 cup of borax
- 1 bar of natural soap
- 2 to 3 teaspoons of baking soda

Directions:

Grate your soap with a grater, or you can grind it in a food processor. Place your grated soap in large mixing bowl and stir in the washing soda, baking soda, and borax. Store your simple dry laundry detergent in a large container or divide it into smaller containers. Cover it tightly and shake before each use. Use 1/4 cup per load.

5. Citrus & Lavender Laundry Soap

This citrus and lavender soap uses all natural ingredients, leaving your clothing smelling fresh and clean.

Ingredients:

- 1/2 cup of borax

- 1/2 cup of washing soda

- 1/2 bar of Castile, Ivory or other natural soap

- 20 drops of lavender essential oil

- 20 drops of citrus essential oil

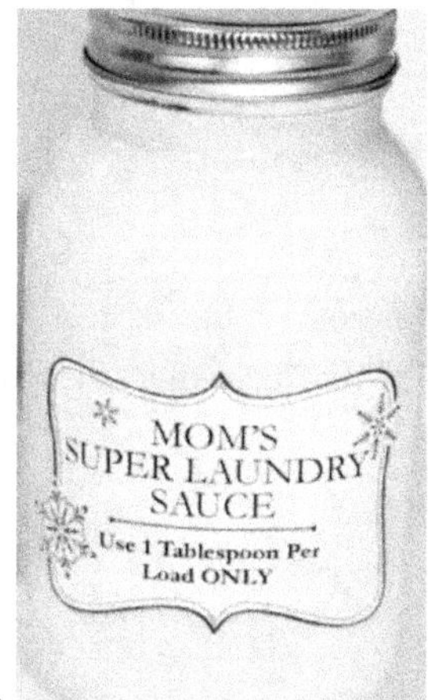

Directions:

Grate your soap in a blender or a food processor, or shred it using a fine grater. Place 4 cups of water in a large pot over medium-low heat. Add in the grated soap, borax and washing soap. Heat the mix while stirring it gently using a wooden spoon. Make sure that the ingredients are all completely dissolved. Remove from heat then add in your essential oils. Pour 2 gallons of hot water into 2 one gallon jugs so that each of them is half full. Using a funnel fill the jugs to the top with soap mixture. Secure lids on jugs and then shake gently. Allow the mixture to settle for 24 hours before using it. Use 1/4 to 1/2 cup of citrus lavender soap per load. Shake gently before using.

6. *Basic Arm & Hammer Laundry Detergent*
Ingredients:

- 3 cups of baking soda

- 1 cup Castile soap

Directions:

Mix these ingredients in a bowl to blend them. There you have it a real simple laundry detergent. The baking soda will help to eliminate odors and stains.

7. Sensitive Skin Detergent
Ingredients:

- 1/4 cup of washing soda

- 1/4 cup of baking soda

- 1/4 cup of sea salt

- 4 ounces bar of soap

- 1/2 cup of white vinegar

- 6 drops of essential oil of your choice

Directions:

Grate your bar of soap and mix the ingredients in a mixing bowl. Add in a bit of vinegar at a time, while you are stirring the mix with a wooden spoon. You want the consistency of it to be clumpy almost like cookie dough. Allow it to sit for 24 hours then it will be ready to use.

8. No-Bake Laundry Detergent

Ingredients:

- 5 ounce bar of natural pure soap

- 1 cup of Arm & Hammer washing soda

- 3 cups of warm water

- 1 cup of Borax powder

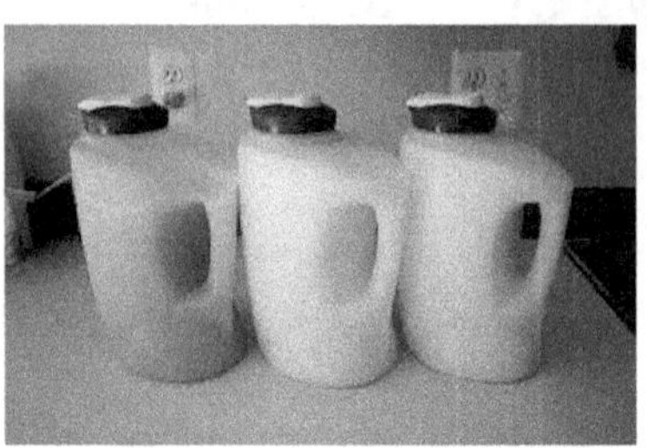

Directions:

Grate up the bar of soap. Divide it up and add to 2 containers. Add in hot water to each container and allow it to set overnight. It is going to look like candle wax in the morning. Cut some indentations into it. Next add in 1/2 cup borax and the same amount of washing soda into each jar or container. Seal the containers. Allow it to sit until smooth. Shake gently before each use. Use one cup per load.

9. *Borax-free Laundry Detergent*

Ingredients:

- 1 cup of washing soda

- 1 bar of Castile soap

- 1/2 cup of baking soda

Directions:

Grate your soap into a mixing bowl. Add in the other ingredients and blend them well. Keep it in an air-tight container. Use 1/4 to 1/2 cup for each load of laundry.

10. Homemade Lemon Liquid Laundry Detergent
Ingredients:

- 1 cup of Borax

- 1 cup of Arm & Hammer washing soda

- 1 bar of pure natural soap

- 20 drops of lemon essential oil

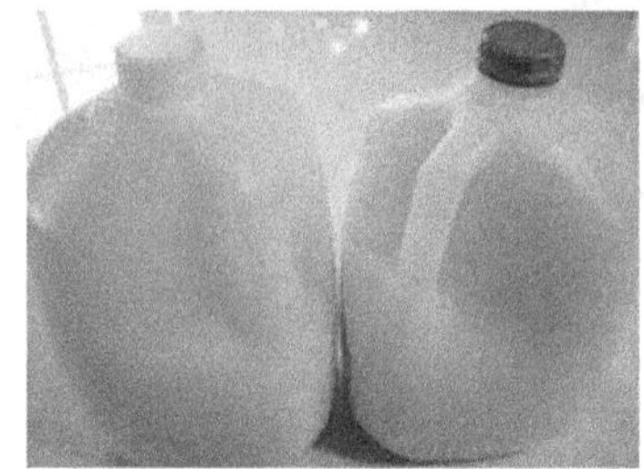

Directions:

Grate up your bar of soap into a mixing bowl. Add it to a pot with 4 cups of boiling water in it. Stir with wooden spoon for about ten minutes or until it is all melted. Have 2 one gallon jugs, fill up halfway with hot water. Pour in the soap mixture, adding in one cup of Arm & hammer washing soda and 1/2 cup of borax. Add in the lemon essential oils. Mix gently. Allow this to set for 24 hours. Shake gently before each use. Use half a cup for each load.

11. *Pine Fresh Laundry Detergent*
Ingredients:

- 1 bar of natural or pure soap

- 1 cup of borax

- 1 cup of Arm & Hammer washing soda

- 20 drops of pine essential oil

Directions

Grate the soap in a mixing bowl. Add in other ingredients and blend well. Use one teaspoon per load of laundry. You will love the fresh pine scent on your clothes!

Homemade Fabric Softeners

12. Citrusy Fabric Softener Sheets

You can replace those expensive unhealthy fabric softener sheets with these wonderful Citrusy fabric softener sheets. Use your old t-shirts to make these sheets.

Ingredients:

- 1/3 cup of white vinegar

- 10 drops of citrus essential oil

- 8 drops of tea tree essential oil

Directions:

Cut your soft fabric such as old t-shirts into 5-inch squares. Place the squares neatly in a plastic container with a secure lid. Measure the white vinegar in a mixing bowl. Stir in the essential oils and blend well. Pour mixture over the fabric in container and seal the lid.

Remove a dryer sheet from container squeezing out any excess liquid before you add the sheet to your dryer. Each of these sheets can be returned to the container to be reused at least three times or until the liquid has been totally absorbed from container. Get a bit adventurous and try different essential oils for your sheets.

_13._ **_Rose Fabric Softener_**

This is an all-natural fabric softener and refresher that is going to effectively neutralize any stubborn odors. Use the cheapest vodka you can find.

Ingredients:

- 1/4 cup of vodka

- 3 cups of white vinegar

- 20 drops of rose essential oil

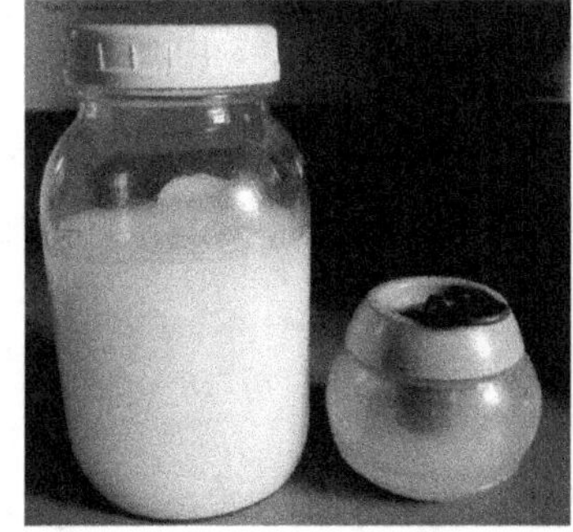

Directions:

Add your ingredients into a container and shake well. Use about 1/2 cup of Rose fabric softener per load.

14. Lavender Fabric Softener

This is a very simple, eco-friendly fabric softener that will leave your laundry feeling and smelling fresh.

Ingredients:

- 3 cups of white vinegar

- 1/2 cup of baking soda

- 20 drops of lavender essential oil

Directions:

In a large mixing bowl add in one cup of water with the baking soda. Mix well. Slowly add in the vinegar and gently stir. Stir in an additional 4 cups of water along with the lavender essential oil. Store in a plastic container with a secure lid. Use one cup of lavender fabric softener in the final rinse cycle, or in your machine's fabric softener dispenser.

15. Fresh Lemon Scent Fabric Softener
Ingredients:

- 1/2 cup of baking soda

- 30 drops of lemon essential oil

- 2 cups of sea salt

Directions:

Mix in large mixing bowl the 2 cups of sea salt along with the lemon essential oil. Blend well then add in the baking soda and gently stir. Place into an air-tight container and that is it!

16. *Suave Rosemary Mint Fabric Softener*
Ingredients:

- One bottle of Suave Rosemary Mint Hair conditioner

- 3 cups of distilled vinegar

- 6 cups of water

Directions:

Add all of your ingredients into an air-tight container. Blend well, and you are ready to use it.

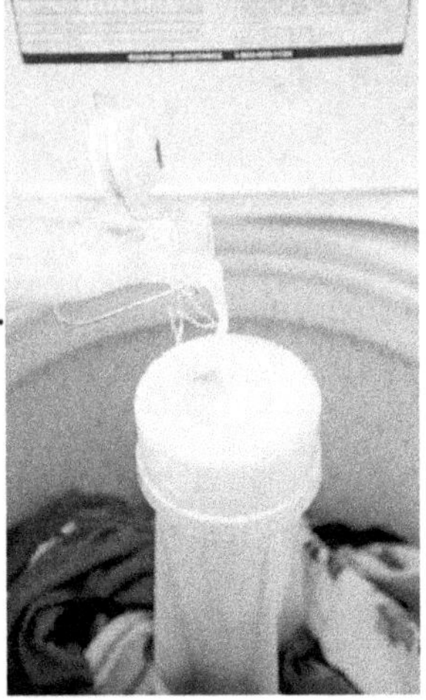

17. Repeat Wash Fabric Softener
Ingredients:

- 4 cups of homemade fabric softener

- 1 large clean towel

Directions:

Take the large towel and soak it in your fabric softener. Place towel over shower curtain rod and allow it to dry. This will leave your house smelling amazing for days! Place the towel into your dryer every time you do a load. Your clothes will come out of the dryer smelling amazing, this will be good for about 30 loads.

Homemade Dryer Sheets

18. Coffee Filter Dryer Sheets
Ingredients:

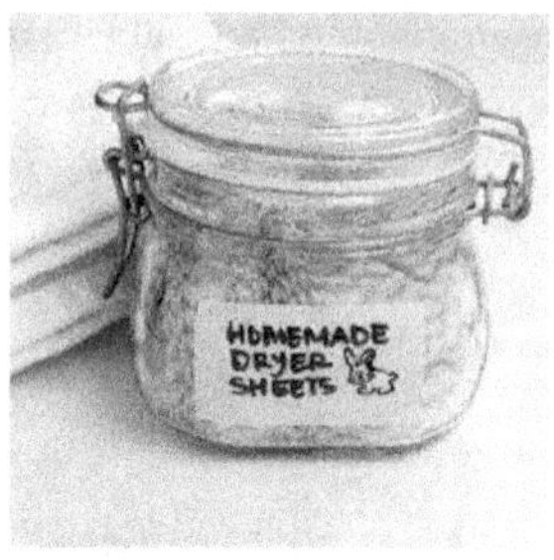

- 1 teaspoon of homemade liquid fabric softener

- 1 coffee filter

Directions:

Pour the softener over the coffee filter. This is a per load recipe. You can probably use one of these for 3 loads.

19. Sweat Stain Remover
Ingredients:

- 1/2 teaspoon of dish detergent

- 1/4 tablespoon of white vinegar

- 1/2 cup of hot water

Directions:

Stir and blend ingredients. Using a small sponge to blot, do not scrub on stained area.

20. Chocolate Stain Remover
Ingredients:

- cold water

- 1/2 cup of baking soda

Directions:

Mix water and baking soda in sink, blot from the
back of stain, using cold water.

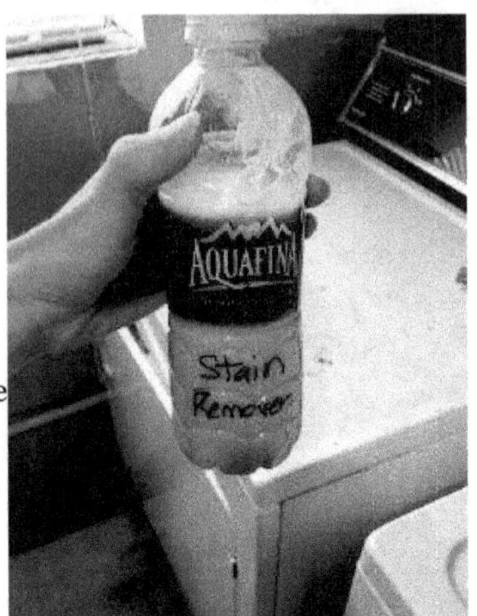

21. Coffee Stain Remover
Ingredients:

- 1/2 teaspoon of white vinegar

- 2 cups of cold water

- sponge

Directions:

Blot vinegar onto stained area then wash in cold water.

22. Red Wine Stain Remover
Ingredients:

- 1 tablespoon of white wine

- 2 teaspoons of sea salt

Directions:

Apply the white wine to the stained area, add a generous amount of sea salt and scrub and rinse immediately.

23. *Makeup or Grease Stain Remover*
Ingredients:

- 3 teaspoons of white vinegar

- 1 teaspoon of baking soda

- cold water

Directions:

Use these ingredients as a pre-wash treatment then
wash as usual.

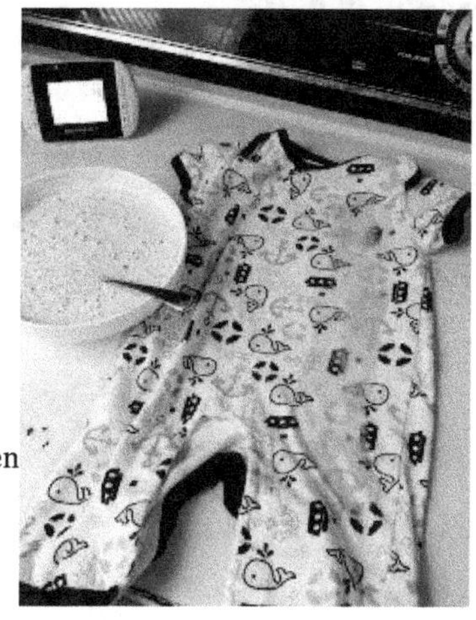

24. Ink Stain Remover
Ingredients:

- Aerosol hairspray

- cold water

Directions:

Spray the hairspray on the stain and rub gently, then run it under cold water.

25. Blood Stain Remover
Ingredients:

- 2 cups of cold water

- 2 teaspoons of sea salt

- 1 teaspoon of ammonia

Directions:

Soak the blood stain in the above ingredients overnight. Next day wash as usual.

26. Terry Cloth & Towel Refresher
Ingredients:

- 1 cup of white vinegar

- 1/2 cup of baking soda

Directions:

When washing your towels and terry cloth items set machine to hot adding in 1 cup of vinegar and 1/2 cup of baking soda. Dry them as usual and they will turn out nice and fluffy just like new!

27. Linen Fabric Spray
Ingredients:

- 10 drops of Eucalyptus essential oil

- 2 cups of distilled water

- 4 drops of chamomile essential oil

- 2 drops of lemon essential oil

Directions:

Add all of your ingredients into a spray bottle and shake well before each use. You can spray this on your clean linens after they have come out of the dryer or before. It is a great fabric spray to use just after making the beds too!

28. Linen Laundry Booster
Ingredients:

- 1 teaspoon of dried orange zest

- 1/2 cup of baking soda

- 1/2 cup of cornstarch

- 10 drops of lemon essential oil

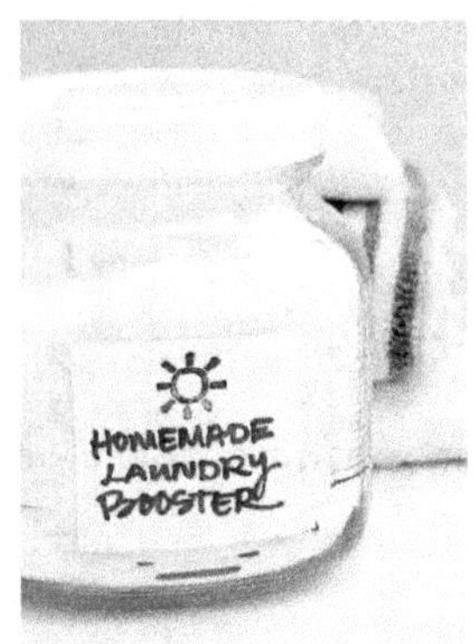

Directions:

Mix all of the ingredients in your blender, then pour into a shaker. Spray or sprinkle on your sheets, comforters etc. Apply before you begin wash.

29. Rose Essential Oil Scent Booster
Ingredients:

- 20 drops of rose essential oil

- 1 pint of white vinegar

- 1/2 a cup of dried rose petals

Directions:

Mix the ingredients and seal in container for about 6 weeks. After this you then need to strain mix to remove any solids left from the pedals. You can use 1/4 to 1/2 cup per load of laundry.

30. Gum Remover from Clothing
Ingredients:

- ice cubes

Directions:

Add ice cubes around where the gum is stuck on article of clothing and let the ice freeze the gum. Once the gum has frozen it should easily break off—and there you have another quick and easy fix!

Conclusion

I hope that you and your loved ones will enjoy using these tips, suggestions and easy to follow laundry detergent recipes. I am sure you will be delighted at the results that you will get in using this wonderful collection of homemade natural chemical-free laundry products. Not to mention you are certain to enjoy the savings you will gain when you stop buying expensive commercial laundry detergents and replace them with your own homemade laundry detergents and other homemade products. There is certainly many benefits to making your own homemade natural cleaning products, but one of the most important benefits is that these are eco-friendly homemade laundry products. You can feel good when you are using your homemade laundry detergent knowing that you are doing your part to help keep the environment safe. Try to spread the good word to others such as friends and family by encouraging them too to start making their own homemade laundry detergents. The best way to show them is by setting an example—show them how well your homemade laundry detergent works and point out the financial savings too!

Thanks again for downloading my book, your support of my work means a great deal to me. I would love to read your review of this book on Amazon. Take care and keep thinking "green" cleaning products—that is the right way to go!

FREE Bonus Reminder

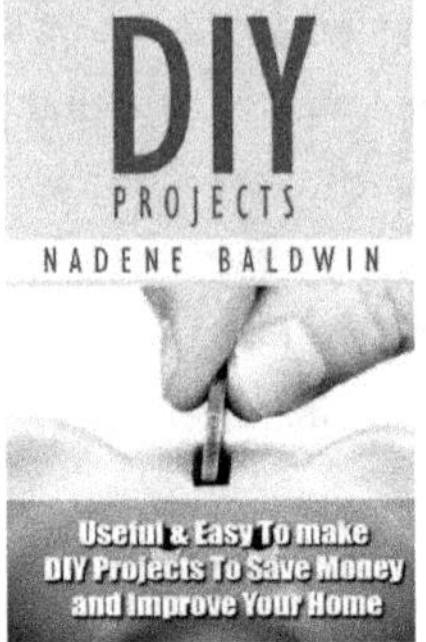

If you have not grabbed it yet, please go ahead and download your special bonus report *"DIY Projects. 13 Useful & Easy To Make DIY Projects To Save Money & Improve Your Home!"*
Simply Click the Button Below

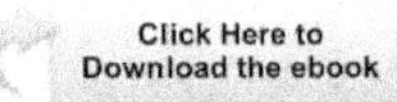

OR **Go to This Page**
http://diyhomecraft.com/free

BONUS #2: More Free & Discounted Books or Products
Do you want to receive more Free/Discounted Books or Products?
We have a mailing list where we send out our new Books or Products when they go free or with a discount on Amazon. Click on the link below to sign up for Free & Discount Book & Product Promotions.
=> Sign Up for Free & Discount Book & Product Promotions <=

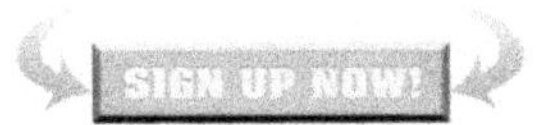

OR Go to this URL
http://zbit.ly/1WBb1Ek